Keto Di

Easy Low-Carb Recipes for Weight Loss

Kimberly Thayer

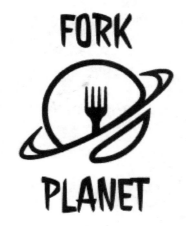

Also by Kimberly Thayer

Kimberly Thayer Keto Cookbooks
Keto Diet Cookbook: Easy Low-Carb Recipes for Weight Loss
Keto Diet Cookbook for Beginners: Simple Low-Carb Recipes for Everyday
Meals

Table of Contents

Introduction

A low-carbohydrate diet is referred to as ketogenic. Protein and fat are intended to provide more calories than carbs. Sugar, soda, pastries, and white bread are simple to digest carbohydrates to eliminate. Your body runs out of fuel rapidly if you consume fewer than 50 grams of carbohydrates each day. In most cases, this process takes three to four days. After then, your body will begin to use protein and fat as a source of energy, which might result in weight loss. This metabolic state is known as ketosis. It's critical to remember that the ketogenic diet is a temporary weight reduction strategy rather than a long-term approach to health. However, a ketogenic diet may also assist medical disorders like epilepsy if used for weight loss alone. Patients with heart problems, some brain illnesses and even acne may get some benefit from it as well.

Unsaturated fats are allowed on the ketogenic diet, such as those found in nuts (walnuts, almonds), seeds (including pumpkin seeds), tofu, avocados, and olive oil. However, oils (coconut, palm), butter, lard, and cocoa butter all contain significant amounts of saturated fats. As a result of the keto diet's high reliance on protein, it does not distinguish between lean and fatty sources of the nutrient. How about fruits and vegetables? However, if you limit your intake to just one or two serves a day, you can get the benefits of some types of fruits (generally berries). Celery and leafy greens are the only vegetables that are rich in carbohydrates. When broccoli is cut into a cup, it has around six grams of carbohydrates.

This cookbook series includes some amazing recipes, prepared using some of the best healthy ingredients. All recipes are created by adding a few extra touches.

The dishes presented in this book are aimed at all members of the family and include everything from breakfast to lunch, snacks to dessert, and mouthwatering dinners. Enjoy!

1. Green Smoothie

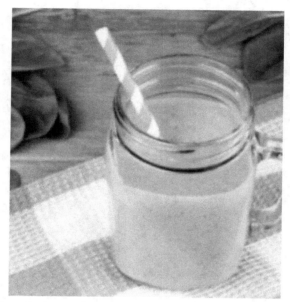

Preparation Time: 5mins
Cooking Time: 0mins
Total time: 5mins
Serves: 1

Ingredients:

- 1 scoop of Whey Protein Jarrow Formulas
- 2 cups of spinach
- 2 brazil nuts
- 10 almonds
- 1 scoop of Greens Powder Amazing Grass
- 1 cup of unsweetened coconut milk

- 1 tbsp of potato starch

Method:
Add first 4 ingredients in blender and blend until they turn smooth. Add rest of the ingredients and blend again.
Tip: Add 1 tbsp of psyllium husk before serving. Enjoy!

Nutrition:
Calories: 380
Fat: 30g
Carbs: 13g
Protein: 12g

2. Chocolate Green Smoothie

Preparation Time: 5mins
Cooking Time: 0mins
Total time: 5mins
Serves: 2

Ingredients:

- 1/4 cup of cocoa powder
- 1/2 cup of frozen berries
- 100 g of spinach chopped
- 1 cup of coconut cream
- 1 tbsp of granulated sweetener

Method:
Add all the ingredients to a blender and blend until you get a thick and smooth mixture. Pour in a glass and serve.
Tip: Adjust the amount of sweetener as per your liking. Enjoy!

Nutrition:
Calories: 362
Fat: 33. 5g
Carbs: 7.6g
Protein: 7.5g

3. Almond Milk Smoothie

Preparation Time: 2 minutes
Cooking Time: 0mins
Total time: 2mins
Serves: 5

Ingredients:

- 1/4 cup of Besti Allulose Powdered
- 1 lb of Frozen strawberries
- 1 Avocado
- 1 1/2 cups of Almond Milk Almond Breeze

Method:
Add all the ingredients to a blender and blend until you get a smooth and creamy texture. Pour and serve in glasses.
Tip: Adjust sweetener as per your liking. Enjoy!

Nutrition:
Calories: 106
Fat: 7g
Carbs: 12g
Protein: 1g

4. Celery Matcha Smoothie

Preparation Time: 5mins
Cooking Time: 0mins
Total time: 5mins
Serves: 1

Ingredients:

- 1 tsp of matcha powder
- 1 baby cucumber
- 1/2 cup of cashew milk
- 1/2 avocado1 stalk of celery
- 1 Tbsp of coconut oil Sweetener

Method:
Add all the ingredients to a blender and blend until you get a smooth and creamy texture. Pour and serve in glasses.
Tip: Adjust amount of sweetener as per your taste. Enjoy!

Nutrition:
Calories: 278
Fat: 27g
Carbs: 12g
Protein: 3g

5. Banana Protein Shake

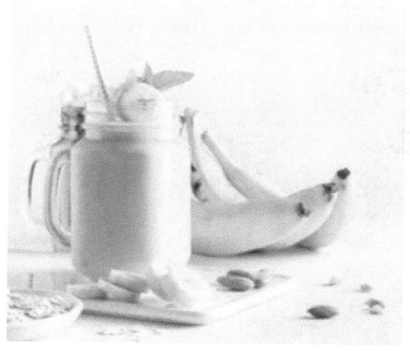

Preparation Time: 10mins
Cooking Time: 0mins
Total time: 10mins
Serves: 1

Ingredients:

Peanut butter protein shake:

- 1 banana, mashed

- 1 cup of almond milk
- 1 tbsp of peanut butter
- 1 scoop of protein powder whey

Method:
Add all the ingredients to a blender and blend until you get a smooth and creamy texture. Pour and serve in glasses.
Tip: You can prepare it up to 3 days in advance and store it in the fridge. Enjoy!

Nutrition:
Calories: 208
Fat: 5g
Carbs: 7g
Protein: 30g

6. Western Omelet

Preparation Time: 5mins
Cooking Time: 25mins
Total time: 30mins
Serves: 2

Ingredients:

- 1/2 chopped green bell pepper
- Eggs
- 2 tbsp of Heavy whipping cream
- Salt & pepper
- 3 oz Shredded cheese
- 2 oz of Butter
- 5 oz of Smoked diced deli ham
- 1/2 chopped yellow onion

Method:
Whisk the eggs and the cream in a mixing dish until moist. Then put salt & pepper. Mix in half the melted cheese and combine properly. Melt the butter over moderate flame in a frying pan. For a couple of minutes, whisk in the sliced ham, onion & peppers. Be extra mindful of not burning the corners. Reduce flame a little bit later. If necessary, fold the omelet.
Tip: Sprinkle with grated cheese before serving. Enjoy!

Nutrition:
Calories: 687

Fat:56g
Carbs: 6g
Protein:40g

7. Pink Drink

Preparation Time: 5mins
Cooking Time: 5mins
Total time: 10mins
Serves: 2

Ingredients:

- 1 tsp of Vanilla Extract
- Two teabags of Fruit Tea Passion
- 1/2 cup of Coconut Cream
- 1 cup of Hot Water
- 2 tbsp of Erythritol
- 1/2 cup of Strawberries quarteredIce to serve

Method:
Steep both the tea bags in hot water in a cup of. Fill 2 glasses with ice. Divide tea among them and whip vanilla extract, erythritol and coconut cream for around 3 minutes with an electric blender. Scoop of over tea and top with strawberries. Tip: Place in fridge for around 15 minutes to chill properly. Enjoy!

Nutrition:
Calories: 123
Fat: 10g
Carbs: 5g
Protein: 2g

8. Milkshake

Preparation Time: 5mins
Cooking Time: 0mins
Total time: 5mins
Serves: 2

Ingredients:

- 1/4 tsp of Ground Ginger
- 1/2 cup of Almond Milk
- 1 cup of canned Coconut Cream
- 1 tsp of Vanilla Extract
- 1 tsp of Erythritol
- 1/2 tsp of Cinnamon
- 1/2 tsp of Turmeric

Method:
Heat coconut cream with almond milk in a pan over low flame. Dissolve rest of the ingredients and stir. Pour into a cup and serve hot.
Tip: You can substitute almond milk with plant-based sugar-free milk. Enjoy!

Nutrition:
Calories: 271
Fat: 24. 7g
Carbs: 2. 2g
Protein: 2.9g

9. Tasty Mexican Breakfast

Preparation Time: 10mins
Cooking Time: 30mins
Total time: 40mins
Serves: 8

Ingredients:

- 1 pitted avocado peeled & chopped
- 1/2 cup of enchilada sauce
- 1 pound ground pork
- 1 pound chopped chorizo
- Salt & black pepper as per taste
- 8 eggs1 chopped tomato
- 3 tbsp of ghee
- 1/2 cup of chopped red onion

Method:
Mix chorizo and pork in a bowl and layer on a baking sheet. Bake in oven for around 20 minutes at 350 °F. Warm ghee in a pan and add eggs. Scramble them and transfer pork to a plate. Top with eggs and add rest of the ingredients on top.
Tip: Top with enchilada sauce to make it even tastier. Enjoy!

Nutrition:
Calories: 400
Fat: 32g

Carbs: 7g
Protein: 25g

10. Cheese & Oregano Muffins

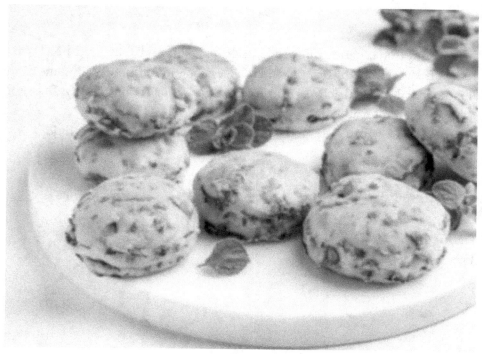

Preparation Time: 10mins
Cooking Time: 25mins
Total time: 35mins
Serves: 6

Ingredients:

- 1 cup of grated cheddar cheese
- 2 tbsp of olive oil
- 1 egg

- 2 tbsp of parmesan cheese
- 1/2 tsp of dried oregano
- 1 cup of almond flour
- 1/4 tsp of baking soda
- Salt & black pepper as per taste
- 1/2 cup of coconut milk

Method:
Mix baking soda, parmesan, pepper, salt, oregano and flour in a bowl. Mix rest of the ingredients except cheddar cheese in another bowl. Combine both mixtures and mix. Stir cheddar in mixture and pour in muffin tray. Bake for around 25 minutes at 350 °F.
Tip: Wait for a few minutes to let the muffins settle before serving. Enjoy!

Nutrition:
Calories: 160
Fat: 3g
Carbs: 6g
Protein: 10g

11. Protein Coffee

Preparation Time: 5mins
Cooking Time: 0mins
Total time: 5mins
Serves: 1

Ingredients

- 1 scoop of protein powder of choice
- 6 oz of brewed coffee
- 2 tbsp of heavy whipping cream
- 1 tbsp of coconut oil
- 1 tbsp of cacao powder

Method:
Mix everything in a mug and use an immersion blender to get a smooth mixture.
Tip: Use cacao powder for the chocolaty taste. Enjoy!

Nutrition:
Calories: 342
Fat: 26g
Carbs: 4g
Protein: 27g

12. Almond Crusted Cheesecake

Preparation Time: 20mins
Cooking Time: 45mins
Total time: 1 hour and 5mins
Serves: 24

Ingredients

Crust:

- 2 tbsp of Sweetener Joy-Filled
- 2 cups of whole almonds
- 4 tbsp of salted butter

Filling:

- ¾ cup of Sweetener Joy-Filled
- 1/2 tsp of vanilla extract
- 16 oz of cottage cheese 4% fat
- 6 eggs
- 8 oz of cream cheese
- 1/2 tsp of almond extract

Topping when serving:

- 1/4 cup of frozen berries mixed, thawed per cheesecake

Method:
Preheat your oven to 350°F. Pulse crust ingredients in a blender and oil 2 muffin pans with 12 holes each. Divide dough among holes and press. Bake for around 8 minutes. Pulse cottage and cream cheese in blender and add extracts and sweetener. Blend again. Add eggs and blend once more. Divide mixture into cups and bake for around 40 minutes. Serve with frozen berries after thawing them.

Tip: If you did not use silicon cups, refrigerate the cups for around 2 hours before trying to take them out. Enjoy!

Nutrition:
Calories: 152
Fat: 12g
Carbs: 3g
Protein: 6g

13. Egg Loaf

Preparation Time: 10mins
Cooking Time: 50mins
Total time: 1 hour
Serves: 12

Ingredients:

- 4 tbsp of melted butter unsalted
- 8 Eggs
- 1/2 cup of Coconut Flour
- 8 oz of full-fat Cream Cheese
- 1 tsp of Baking Powder

Method:

Preheat your oven to 350 °F. Mix eggs with cream cheese and butter in a bowl. Fold in the coconut flour and baking powder. Pour mixture into a loaf pan. Bake for around 50 minutes.

Tip: Line the pan usin g parchment paper before pourin g the mixture. Enjoy!

Nutrition:
Calories: 177
Fat: 14.2g
Carbs: 6.8g
Protein: 6.3g

14. Zucchini Hash Browns

Preparation Time: 15mins
Cooking Time: 30mins
Total time: 45mins
Serves: 2

Ingredients:

- 1/8 cup of Butter
- 1.5 lb of Zucchini
- 2 Eggs
- 1/2 tsp of Salt
- 2 cloves of minced Garlic
- 1/4 cup of grated Parmesan Cheese

Method:
Shred zucchini in a bowl and add salt. Leave for around 15 minutes. Squeeze extra moisture and add garlic, cheese and eggs. Warm 2 tbsp of butter in a pan and mound 2 tbsp of mixture in pan and flatten it to make a patty. Cook each side for around 3 minutes and repeat with all the mixture.
Tip: You can add more butter to pan if that is required. Enjoy!

Nutrition:
Calories: 270
Fat: 20g
Carbs: 11g
Protein: 14. 5g

15. Mini Crustless Quiches

Preparation Time: 15mins
Cooking Time: 25mins
Total time: 40mins
Serves: 6

Ingredients:

- 1/3 cup of Heavy Cream
- 14 Eggs
- 2/3 cup of Mozzarella Cheese diced into tiny pieces
- 3 diced Plum Tomatoes
- 1/3 cup of diced White Onion
- 1/3 cup of grated Cheddar Cheese
- 2/3 cup of Salami diced
- 1/3 cup of sliced Pickled Jalapenos

Method:
Preheat your oven to 320°F. Add all the ingredients to a bowl and season with pepper and salt. Mix and divide among muffin tins equally. Bake for around 25 minutes.

Tip: You can serve it right away or store it in fridge and reheat it for later use. Enjoy!

Nutrition:
Calories: 270
Fat: 30g

Carbs: 6g
Protein: 26g

16. Waffle Breakfast Sandwich

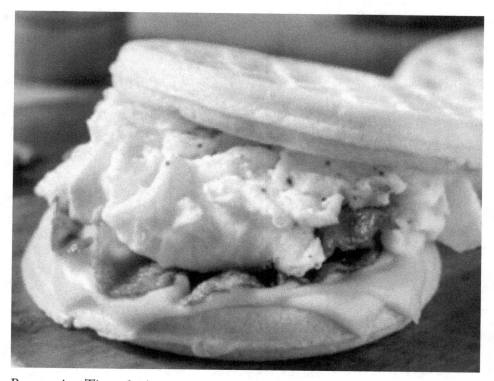

Preparation Time: 1min
Cooking Time: 8min
Total time: 9min
Serves: 1

Ingredients:

- 2 tbsp of butter
- 1egg

- 1 tbsp of almond flour
- 1/2 cup of Monterey cheese

Method:

Mix egg, Monterey cheese and almond flour in a bowl. Pour half the mixture and cook for around 4 minutes. Repeat with the rest of the mixture. Melt butter in a pan and cook each side of waffles for around 2 minutes.

Tip: Serve with fruit on the side. Enjoy!

Nutrition:

Calories: 514

Fat: 47g

Carbs: 2g

Protein: 14g

17. Ranch Chicken

Preparation Time: 3mins
Cooking Time: 22mins
Total time: 25mins
Serves: 4

Ingredients:

- 1/4 cup scallions, chopped
- 2 chicken breasts
- 2 tbsp of butter, melted
- 1 tsp of salt
- 1/2 tsp of garlic powder
- 1/2 tsp of cayenne pepper
- 1/2 tsp of black peppercorns, crushed
- 1/2 tbsp of ranch seasoning mix
- 4 ounces Ricotta cheese, room temperature
- 1/2 cup Monterey-Jack cheese, grated
- 4 slices bacon, chopped

Method:
Preheat the oven to 370°F. Drizzle butter over chicken. Add seasonings to chicken and cook chicken in the pan for around 5 minutes on each side. Coat a baking dish and add chicken. Add bacon and cheese and bake for around 12 minutes. Add scallions on top.
Tip: Sprinkle some grated cheese on top before serving. Enjoy!

Nutrition:
Calories: 295
Fat: 19. 5g
Carbs: 2.9g
Protein: 3.1g

18. Butter bread

Preparation Time: 5mins
Cooking Time: 55mins
Total time: 1 hour
Serves: 20

Ingredients:

Bread:

- 3 eggs, only whites
- 11/4 cups of almond flour
- 5 tbsp of psyllium husk ground
- 2 tsp of baking powder
- 1 tsp of sea salt
- 1 cup of water
- 2 tsp of cider vinegar

Garlic butter:

- 1/2 tsp of salt
- 4 oz. of butter
- 1 minced garlic clove
- 2 tbsp of chopped fresh parsley

Method:
Preheat oven to around 350°F. Line parchment paper on the baking sheet and
mix dry ingredients in a bowl. Boil water and add egg whites, vinegar and water

to dry ingredients. Whisk for around 30 seconds. Roll into hot dog-shaped buns and place them on a sheet. Bake for around 40 minutes. Mix ingredients for garlic butter and refrigerate. Cut buns from the center and spread butter. Bake for 15 minutes at 425°F.

Tip: Glaze with 1 tbsp of melted butter on top at the end. Enjoy!

Nutrition:
Calories: 91
Fat: 8g
Carbs: 1g
Protein: 2g

19. Cranberry Bread

Preparation Time: 20mins
Cooking Time: 60mins
Total time: 1 hour and 20mins
Serves: 12

Ingredients:

- 6 ounces of cranberries
- 1 1/2 cups of almond flour
- 1/2 cup of white sweetener
- 1/2 cup of almond milk unsweetened
- 1/2 cup of coconut flour
- 1/2 tsp of 30% extract monk fruit
- 1 1/2 tsp of baking powder
- 1 tbsp of orange peel dried
- 1/2 tsp of baking soda
- 1/2 tsp of ground cinnamon
- 1/2 tsp of xanthan gum
- 1/2 tsp of salt
- 1/4 cup of butter melted
- 1/4 tsp of ground nutmeg
- 6 eggs

Method:
Preheat oven to around 325°F. Oil a pan and line using parchment paper.
Mix everything except butter, egg and almond milk in a bowl. Mix them in

a separate bowl. Add to dry ingredients and whisk. Fold the mixture in cranberries and pour in a pan. Bake for around 1 hour.

Tip: Use unsalted butter for the best results. Enjoy!

Nutrition:
Calories: 175
Fat: 14g
Carbs: 8g
Protein: 7g

20. Greek-Style Frittata with Herbs

Preparation Time: 5mins
Cooking Time: 25mins
Total time: 30mins
Serves: 4

Ingredients

- 4 ounces of crumbled Feta cheese
- 6 eggs
- 1/2 cup of heavy cream
- 2 tbsp of yogurt Greek-style
- 2 ounces of chopped bacon
- Sea salt & ground black pepper as per taste
- 1 tbsp of olive oil
- 1/2 cup of peeled red onions sliced
- 1 chopped garlic clove
- 8 pitted Kalamata olives sliced
- 1 tsp of dried oregano
- 1/2 tsp of dried rosemary
- 1/2 tsp of dried marjoram

Method:
Preheat the oven to 360°F. Spray a baking pan using cooking spray and mix pepper, salt, bacon, yogurt, cream and eggs in a bowl. Warm oil in a pan and cook garlic and onion for around 3 minutes. Transfer to baking pan and pour mixture of eggs on top. Add rest of the ingredients except feta cheese and bake

for around 13 minutes. Scatter cheese on top and bake for 3 more minutes.
Tip: Let it settle for around 5 minutes before cutting into pieces and serving.
Enjoy!

Nutrition:
Calories: 345
Fat: 28.5g
Carbs: 4.4g
Protein: 18. 2g

21. Healthy Pumpkin Bars

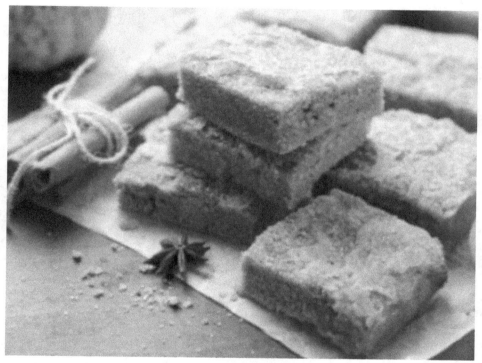

Preparation Time: 10mins
Cooking Time: 20mins
Total time: 30mins
Serves: 1

Ingredients:

- 1/2 tsp of Vanilla Extract
- 1/2 cup of Flaked Coconut
- 1/2 cup of Sunflower Seeds

- 1/4 cup of Sliced Almonds
- 2/3 cup of Almond Flour
- 1 Egg
- 1/4 cup of Pumpkin Puree
- 1/4 cup of Coconut Oil
- 1 1/2 tsp of Baking Powder
- 1/4 cup of Erythritol
- 2/3 tsp of Pumpkin Pie Spice
- 1/4 tsp of Salt

Method:
Preheat the oven to 325°F. Process sunflower seeds and coconut oil in a blender. Mix rest of the ingredients in another bowl and add the prepared puree. Spread on the pan and bake for around 20 minutes.
Tip: Use a 9x9' baking pan of square shape for this recipe for best results. Enjoy!

Nutrition:
Calories: 153
Fat: 13.3g
Carbs: 12g
Protein: 3.2g

22. Cloud bread

Preparation Time: 5mins
Cooking Time: 25mins
Total time: 30mins
Serves: 2

Ingredients:

- 1/2 tsp of baking powder
- 3 eggs
- 1 pinch of salt
- 4 oz. of cream cheese
- 1/2 tbsp of psyllium husk ground
- 1/4 tsp of cream of tartar

Method:

Preheat oven to around 300°F. Add egg yolks to one bowl and whites to another. Mix salt in whites and add the rest of the ingredients to yolks. Mix two bowls and place them on a baking tray lined with paper. Spread into circles and bake for around 25 minutes.

Tip: Sprinkle chopped nuts on top. Enjoy!

Nutrition:
Calories: 740
Fat: 61g
Carbs: 7g
Protein: 37g

23. Spinach Stuffed Chicken Breasts

Preparation Time: 15mins
Cooking Time: 10mins
Total time: 25mins
Serves: 6

Ingredients:

- 1 tsp of Olive oil
- 3 Chicken breasts
- 8 oz Spinach cooked chopped frozen
- 3 oz Feta crumbled
- 4 oz of Cream cheese
- 1 clove Diced garlic
- 1/4 tsp of Salt
- 1/8 tsp of Pepper

Method:
Preheat the oven to 440°F. In a medium bowl, combine the sliced frozen spinach, feta, cream, garlic & half the salt. Slice chicken breast into a pocket. Separate the spinach & cheese combination into 3 parts & roll into thinner logs. Stuff every log into the chicken breast pocket you've made. Sprinkle with salt & pepper. In an oven-proof pan placed over high flame, warm the olive oil, after which apply the stuffed chicken, side down "row. " cook for five min, after this turn over the chicken. Place the frying pan in the oven and cook for around 10 minutes. If the chicken breasts are exceptionally thinner, cook for around 5 minutes more.

Tip: Sprinkle with some grated cheese before serving. Enjoy!

Nutrition:
Calories: 434
Fat: 16g
Carbs: 3g
Protein: 6g

24. Chicken Enchilada

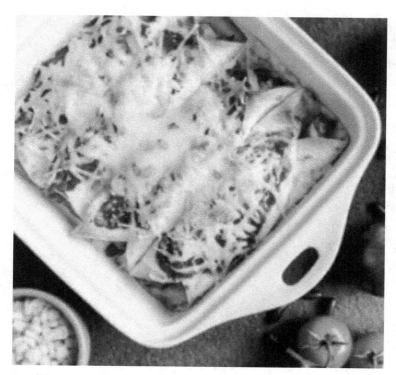

Preparation Time: 25mins
Cooking Time: 20mins
Total time: 45mins
Serves: 1

Ingredients:

- 1/4 cup of Sour cream
- 20 oz Frozen cauliflower florets
- 4 oz of Softened cream cheese

- 2 cups of shredded cooked chicken
- 1/2 cup of Salsa Verde
- 1/2 tsp of Kosher salt
- 1/8 tsp of ground black pepper
- 1 cup of Cheddar cheese shredded

Method:
Place the cauliflower in a safe microwave plate and bake for around 12 minutes or till the pork is soft. Before you microwave for another thirty secs, add the cream cheese. Stir in the chicken, green salsa, pepper, salt, sour cream, cilantro& cheddar cheese. Bake for 20 minutes inside an oven-proof baking dish in a preheated oven at 374 °F.
Tip: Sprinkle with some grated cheese before serving. Enjoy!

Nutrition:
Calories: 311
Fat: 18g
Carbs: 4g
Protein: 33g

25. Fennel and Chicken Lunch Salad

Preparation Time: 10mins
Cooking Time: 0min
Total time: 10mins
Serves: 4

Ingredients:

- A pinch of cayenne pepper
- 3 boneless & skinless chicken breasts, cooked & chopped
- 2 tbsp of walnut oil
- 1/4 cup of toasted walnuts chopped
- 1 & 1/2 cup of chopped fennel
- 2 tbsp of lemon juice
- 1/4 cup of mayonnaise
- 2 tbsp of chopped fennel fronds
- Salt & black pepper as per taste

Method:
Mix walnuts, chicken and fennel in a bowl. Mix rest of the ingredients in another bowl. Pour chicken over the other mixture and toss.
Tip: Serve right away or store in fridge until ready to serve. Enjoy!

Nutrition:
Calories: 200
Fat: 10g
Carbs: 3g

Protein: 7g

26. Delicious Broccoli Soup

Preparation Time: 10mins
Cooking Time: 30mins
Total time: 40mins
Serves: 4

Ingredients:

- 1/2 tsp of paprika
- 1 chopped white onion
- 1 tbsp of ghee
- 2 cups of veggie stock
- Salt & black pepper as per taste
- 2 cups of water
- 2 minced garlic cloves
- 1 cup of heavy cream
- 8 ounces of grated cheddar cheese
- 12 ounces of broccoli florets

Method:
Warm ghee in a pan and stir cook garlic and ghee for around 5 minutes. Add rest of the ingredients except cheese and broccoli and stir. Boil and stir broccoli in mixture. Simmer for around 25 minutes. Blend in a blender and add cheese. Blend once more and serve.
Tip: You can omit the cheese if you feel like this sounds a bit too heavy for your diet. Enjoy!

Nutrition:
Calories: 350
Fat: 34g
Carbs: 7g
Protein: 11g

27. Caprese Salad

Preparation Time: 5mins
Cooking Time: 0min
Total time: 5mins
Serves: 2

Ingredients:

- 1 tbsp of olive oil
- 1/2 pound of sliced mozzarella cheese
- 1 sliced tomato
- Salt & black pepper as per taste
- 4 torn basil leaves
- 1 tbsp of balsamic vinegar

Method:
Add mozzarella slices on one plate and tomato on another plate. Sprinkle with pepper and salt and drizzle olive oil and vinegar. Sprinkle leaves on top and serve.
Tip: Sprinkle some shredded cheese on top of both plates before serving. Enjoy!

Nutrition:
Calories: 150
Fat: 12g
Carbs: 6g
Protein: 9g

28. Rye Waffles

Preparation Time: 2mins
Cooking Time: 4mins
Total time: 6mins
Serves: 1

Ingredients:

- 1/2 tsp of baking powder
- 1egg
- 1/2 tsp of caraway seeds
- 1 tbsp of melted butter
- 2 tbsp of almond flour
- 1 tbsp of mozzarella cheesepinch of garlic powderpinch of salt

Method:
Add all the ingredients to a bowl and mix. Pour half amount of mixture into the maker and cook for around 4 minutes. Repeat with the rest of the mixture. Tip: Sprinkle cheese on top before serving. Enjoy!

Nutrition:
Calories: 263
Fat: 18.8g
Carbs: 10.6g
Protein: 3.1g

29. Belgian Waffles

Preparation Time: 2mins
Cooking Time: 4mins
Total time: 6mins
Serves: 2

Ingredients:

- 2 eggs
- 1.5 cups of shredded jack and cheddar cheese

Method:
Beat eggs in a bowl and add shredded cheese. Mix the cheese in eggs and pour in the maker. Cook for around 4 minutes.
Tip: Sprinkle cheese on top before serving. Enjoy!

Nutrition:
Calories: 300
Fat: 23g
Carbs: 2.6g
Protein: 20g

30. Savory Waffles with Jalapenos and Ham

Preparation Time: 5mins
Cooking Time: 12mins
Total time: 17mins
Serves: 4

Ingredients:

- 1/4 of ham steak
- 2 eggs
- 1 scallion
- 1/2 of jalapeno pepper
- 1/4 cup of cheddar cheese
- 2 tsp of flour, coconut

Method:
Grate the cheese. Shred jalapeno too. Cut scallions and ham. Mix all these ingredients. Pour a quarter of this mixture into the maker and cook for around 2 to 3 minutes until crispy. Repeat the process.
Tip: Sprinkle cheese on top before serving. Enjoy!

Nutrition:
Calories: 119
Fat: 8g
Carbs: 2g
Protein: 10g

31. Garlic Cheesy Waffle Bread Sticks

Preparation Time: 2mins
Cooking Time: 8mins
Total time: 10mins
Serves: 8

Ingredients:

- 1/2 tsp of oregano
- 1 egg
- 2 tbsp of almond flour
- 1/2 cup of grated mozzarella cheese
- 1/2 tsp of garlic powder
- 1/2 tsp of salt

Topping:

- 1/4cup of grated mozzarella cheese
- 1/2 tsp of garlic powder
- 2 tbsp of unsalted butter softened

Method:
Beat eggs in a bowl. Add the rest of the ingredients and mix. Pour the mixture into the maker and cook for around 5 minutes. Make 4 strips of each waffle. Place on a tray and mix garlic powder and butter in a bowl. Spread the mixture over sticks and preheat the grill. Sprinkle sticks with mozzarella and cook under the grill for around 3 minutes.
Tip: Sprinkle cheese on top before serving. Enjoy!

Nutrition:
Calories: 74
Fat: 6.5g
Carbs: 0.9g
Protein: 3.4g

32. Cheesy Zucchini Casserole

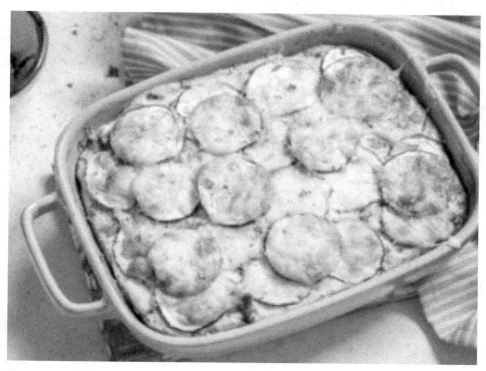

Preparation Time: 5mins
Cooking Time: 45mins
Total time: 50mins
Serves: 4

Ingredients

- 1 tsp of minced garlic
- cooking spray Nonstick
- 2 cups of sliced zucchini

- 2 tbsp of sliced leeks
- 1/2 tsp of salt black pepper ground
- 1/2 tsp of dried basil
- 1/2 tsp of dried oregano
- 1/2 cup of grated Cheddar cheese
- 1/4 cup of heavy cream
- 4 tbsp of grated Parmesan cheese
- 1 tbsp of butter

Method:
Preheat the oven to 370°F. Spray a dish using cooking spray and add 1 cup of zucchini slices to dish. Add 1 tbsp of leeks and sprinkle with seasonings. Top with quarter cup of cheddar cheese. Repeat layers 1 more time and whisk parmesan, garlic, butter and heavy cream in a bowl. Spread over dish mixture and bake in oven for around 45 minutes.
Tip: Sprinkle with chives before serving. Enjoy!

Nutrition:
Calories: 155
Fat: 13g
Carbs: 3.5g
Protein: 7.6g

33. Smoked Haddock Fish Burgers

Preparation Time: 5mins
Cooking Time: 15mins
Total time: 20mins
Serves: 4

Ingredients

- 4 lemon wedges
- 2 tbsp of sunflower oil
- 8 ounces of smoked haddock
- 1 egg
- 1/4 cup of grated Parmesan cheese
- 1 tsp of chili powder
- 1 tsp of parsley flakes dried
- 1/4 cup of chopped scallions
- 1 tsp of minced garlic
- Salt & ground black pepper as per taste

Method:
Warm 1 tbsp of oil in a pan and cook haddock for around 6 minutes. Discard bones and skin and flake them into tiny pieces. Mix rest of the ingredients except oil in a bowl. Warm rest of oil and cook burgers for around 6 minutes. Tip: Garnish using lemon wedges before serving. Enjoy!

Nutrition:
Calories: 174

Fat: 11.4g
Carbs: 1.5g
Protein: 15.4g

34. Zucchini Noodles

Preparation Time: 10mins
Cooking Time: 10mins
Total time: 20mins
Serves: 4

Ingredients

- 1 tbsp of olive oil
- 4 medium-sized zucchinis

Sauce:

- 1/4 cup of sweet chili sauce
- 1/4 cup of fat-free plain Greek yogurt
- 1 1/2 tsp of sriracha sauce
- 2 tsp of lime juice
- 1 1/2 tbsp of honey
- 1/4 cup of light mayonnaise

Method:
Add olive oil to a large skillet, cook the zucchini on medium heat. Add noodles to it. Cook until desired tenderness. Drain the zucchini noodles and let them rest for around 10 minutes. Take a separate bowl, mix all sauce ingredients. Mix the noodles. Keep in fridge for 3 days. Heat up the noodles when you want to eat and add sauce.
Tip: Keep the sauce in containers for later use. Enjoy!

Nutrition:
Calories: 185
Fat: 7.6g
Carbs: 15.5g
Protein: 5. 2g

35. Spicy Avocados

Preparation Time: 10mins
Cooking Time: 0mins
Total time: 10mins
Serves: 4

Ingredients

- 1 tsp of toasted sesame oil
- 1/2 lb. of sushi-grade ahi tuna
- 2 tbsp of mayonnaise
- 2 medium California avocados
- Sea salt as per taste
- Sesame seeds
- 2 tsp of Sriracha sauce

Method:
Cut the tuna finely. Take a bowl, add sesame oil, mayonnaise, Sriracha sauce, and tuna. Mix well. Slice avocados in half to remove pits. Sprinkle some salt over top. Add tuna mixture into avocados and sprinkle sesame seeds over it.
Tip: You can add wasabi if you like sushi. Enjoy!

Nutrition:
Calories: 160
Fat: 17.8g
Carbs: 7. 3g
Protein: 15. 7g

36. Keto Cheeseburger Casserole

Preparation Time: 10mins
Cooking Time: 15mins
Total time: 25mins
Serves: 6

Ingredients

For Beef Layer:

- 1 onion, quartered and sliced
- 1 clove garlic, crushed
- 1.6 lb of ground beef
- Salt/pepper to taste
- 2 oz of cream cheese
- 3 slices of bacon, diced

For Cheese Sauce:

- 1/2 cup grated cheese
- 3 eggs
- 2 pickles, sliced
- 1/2 cup of heavy cream
- 1 cup of shredded cheese
- Salt/pepper to taste
- 2 tbsp of mustard

Method:
Fry bacon pieces and set them aside. Cook beef with onions and garlic. Once it's cooked, add seasonings and cream cheese. Pour beef layer in a dish with bacon on top. For cheese sauce, mix mustard, cream, cheese, salt, eggs and pepper in a bowl. Pour this sauce over beef and bacon layers. Top it with cheese and pickles and bake at 350 °F for about 15 minutes. Serve with sauce and salad. Tip: This casserole is made up of two simple layers. In between each layer, you can get creative and stuff it with all of your preferred fillings, just like you would with a regular cheeseburger. Enjoy!

Nutrition:
Calories: 613.2
Fat: 51.1g
Carbs: 2.9g
Protein: 33. 2g

37. Keto Cordon Bleu Casserole

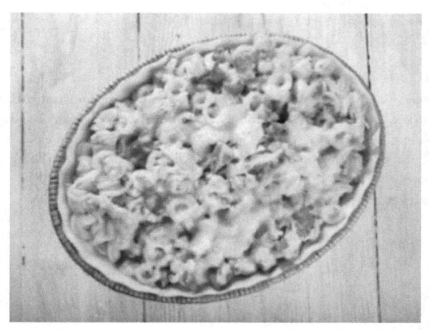

Preparation Time: 20mins
Cooking Time: 55mins
Total time: 1 hour 15mins
Serves: 4

Ingredients:

- 2 large cloves of garlic, crushed
- 4 oz of cream cheese
- 1 lb of zucchini, sliced
- 1 tbsp of unsalted butter
- 1/2 small onion, diced

- 1/8 tsp of black pepper
- 1 cup of chicken bone broth
- 2 tbsp of pork belly, crisped
- 2 tbsp of grated Parmesan
- 2 tbsp of fresh parsley, chopped
- 2 oz of Emmental cheese, shredded
- 1/2 tsp of Worcestershire sauce
- 2 cups of cooked chicken, shredded

Method:
Preheat oven to 375°F. Add butter to a pan and cook onion until softened. Add garlic and cook. Add chicken broth and boil. Mix cream cheese in it and let it cook until it is thick. Add spices and Worcestershire sauce. Add chicken and zucchini to the dish. Top with sauce, pork belly and cheese. Bake for around 45 minutes.

Tip: If you don't like pork belly, you can also add bacon crumbs. Enjoy!

Nutrition:
Calories: 373
Fat: 13g
Carbs: 8g
Protein: 27g

38. Keto Pasta with 3 Ingredients

Preparation Time: 10mins
Cooking Time: 30mins
Total time: 40mins
Serves: 2

Ingredients

- 4 tsp of Gelatin Powder
- Yolks of 2 large Eggs
- 2 cups of shredded Mozzarella Cheese
- 2 tbsp of Cold Water

Method:
Whisk gelatin and cold water. Melt cheese in microwave and whisk. Add yolk in cheese and whisk well. Microwave gelatin and stir. Mix gelatin with cheese mixture. Make a dough. Put oil on two parchment papers and put dough in them. Roll this dough. Freeze for around 30 minutes. Make strips of dough.
Tip: Make sure gelatin and cheese mixture is not thick. Serve with pasta sauce. Enjoy!

Nutrition:
Calories: 181
Fat: 9.5g
Carbs: 1.6g
Protein: 22.7g

39. Soup with Keto Chicken and Mushrooms

Preparation Time: 15mins
Cooking Time: 20mins
Total time: 35mins
Serves: 2

Ingredients

- Salt to taste
- 2 cups of Chicken Stock
- 7 oz. of sliced Chicken Breast
- 4 tbsp of Sesame Oilcup of chopped Fresh Mushrooms
- tbsp of chopped Fresh Parsley
- tbsp of sherry
- Pepper to taste

Method:
Slice chicken. Boil chicken stock in pan and put mushroom and chicken in it. Set aside when completely boiled. Then put sesame oil, sherry, pepper and salt in the soup. Serve.
Tip: You can sprinkle parsley while serving. Enjoy!

Nutrition:
Calories: 399
Fat: 35g
Carbs: 2.9g
Protein: 23g

40. Greek Frittata on a Keto Diet

Preparation Time: 10mins
Cooking Time: 25mins
Total time: 35mins
Serves: 2

Ingredients

- Scallions
- 5 Eggs
- 1/2 tbsp of Olive Oil
- pinch of Pepper
- 1 pinch of salt
- cup of halved Grape Tomatoes
- 1 oz. of Spinach
- oz. of crumbled Feta Cheese sliced

Method:
Preheat oven at 350 F. Oil casserole pan and heat in oven for around 5 minutes. Whisk eggs with pepper and salt in a bowl. Then put scallions, spinach, tomatoes and feta cheese in egg mixture. Cook this mixture in casserole pan for around 30 minutes.
Tip: Do not overcook casserole. Feta cheese should be properly crumbled. Enjoy!

Nutrition:
Calories: 376.5

Fat: 26g
Carbs: 5.8g
Protein: 27.5g

41. Delicious Mexican Lunch

Preparation Time: 10mins
Cooking Time: 20mins
Total time: 30mins
Serves: 4

Ingredients:

- 2 cups of shredded cheddar cheese
- 1/4 cup of chopped cilantro
- 2 pitted avocados peeled and diced into chunks
- 1 tbsp of lime juice
- 1/4 cup of chopped white onion
- 1 tsp of minced garlic
- Salt & black pepper as per taste
- Six cherry tomatoes, diced in quarters
- 1/2 cup of water
- 2-pound of ground beef meat
- 2 cups of sour cream
- 1/4 cup of taco seasoning
- 2 cups of shredded lettuce leaves

Method:
Mix first 7 ingredients in a bowl and place in fridge. Warm a pan and brown beef for around 10 minutes in it. Add water and taco seasoning and stir. Cook for 10 more minutes. Divide among 4 bowls and add avocado mix and sour cream. Add lettuce and cheddar and enjoy.

Tip: Drizzle with cayenne sauce before serving if you prefer. Enjoy!

Nutrition:
Calories: 340
Fat: 30g
Carbs: 3g
Protein: 32g

42. Recipe for Pumpkin Muffins

Preparation Time: 10mins
Cooking Time: 20mins
Total time: 30mins
Serves: 6

Ingredients

- 1/4 tsp of salt
- 4 Eggs
- 2/3 cup of Coconut Flour
- 1/2 cup of melted Butter
- 1/2 cup of Pumpkin Puree
- 2 tsp of Vanilla Extract
- 2 tbsp of sweetener (Erythritol)
- 1 tsp of Baking Powder
- 2 tsp of Ground Cinnamon

Method:
Preheat oven at 350 F. Cover muffin tins with sheet. Mix puree, eggs, vanilla, cinnamon and butter together. Then put erythritol, baking powder and flour in it. Mix well. Put this mixture in muffin tins. Cook for around 20 minutes. Cool and serve.
Tip: Make sure the oven temperature does not burn the muffins. Keep on checking the muffins while baking. Enjoy!

Nutrition:
Calories: 244
Fat: 19. 6g
Carbs: 8.9g
Protein: 5.8g

43. Salad Nicoise de Poulet

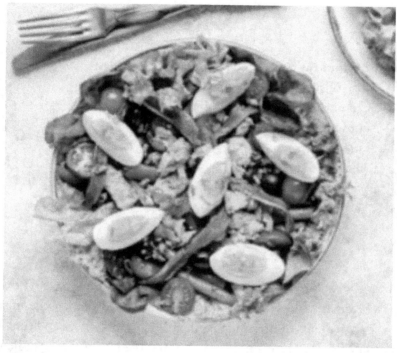

Preparation Time: 10mins
Cooking Time: 20mins
Total time: 30mins
Serves: 4

Ingredients:

- 1/2 lb. of fresh halved green beans

Dressing:

- Dash of pepper
- 2 tsp of lemon zest grated
- 1/4 cup of olive oil
- 2 minced cloves of garlic
- 2 tbsp of lemon juice
- 1/8 tsp of salt
- 1 tsp of Dijon mustard

Salad:

- 1 medium, julienned red pepper
- 2 tbsp of sliced olives
- 1 can of tuna (flaked and drained)
- 2 cups of salad greens, torn and mixed
- 1 tsp of capers
- 1 small, sliced red onion
- 1 package of striped chicken breast, grilled
- 2 hard-boiled chopped eggs (wedges)

Method:
Cook beans in water using a saucepan. When boiled, remove from hot water and keep beans in cold water. Strain and make them dry. In the meantime, mix all the ingredients of dressing together. Mix capers, olives and tuna. Take a plate, put salad greens, tuna mixture, beans and the rest of the ingredients over one another. Serve this with dressing.
Tip: Do not forget to soak beans in cold water. Make even layers of all the ingredients while serving. Enjoy!

Nutrition:
Calories: 289
Fat: 18g
Carbs: 9g
Protein: 24g

44. Ground Beef Pesto Zucchini Stir Fry

Preparation Time: 3mins
Cooking Time: 17mins
Total time: 20mins
Serves: 6

Ingredients:

- 2 tbsp of Fresh chopped parsley
- 1 lb. Ground beef
- 1 tsp of Sea salt
- 1/2 tsp of Black pepper
- 2 Sliced medium Zucchini
- 2 Minced Garlic Cloves
- ¾ c Basil pesto
- 1/2 c Goat cheese

Method:
Cook the minced garlic in a frying pan over medium flame for about a minute until it is fragrant. Add the ground beef. Sprinkle on to taste with salt & pepper. Increase to medium flame. Cook for around 10 minutes until browned, breaking apart with either a spoon or spatula. Add some zucchini. Cook for around 7 minutes, occasionally stirring until the zucchini begins to soften & turn golden. Remove from flame. Add basil pesto. Toss with parsley & goat cheese.

Tip: Sprinkle with some grated cheese before serving. Enjoy!

Nutrition:
Calories: 461
Fat: 36g
Carbs: 9g
Protein: 30.7g

45. Burger Recipe on the Grill or the stovetop

Preparation Time: 5mins
Cooking Time: 8mins
Total time: 13mins
Serves: 4

Ingredients:

- 1/2 tsp of Black pepper
- 1 lb Ground beef
- 1 tbsp of Olive oil
- 1 tbsp of Worcestershire sauce
- 1/2 tsp of Garlic powder
- 1 tsp of Sea salt

Method:
Put in a wide bowl with all ingredients. Function with your hands until you have just packed, taking care not to overwork the meat. Form the patties into 1/2 in (1 cm) wide, around 1/4 pound each. Create a thumbprint in patty's middle to prevent the burgers from bubbling out while frying. Preheat to medium-high grill or skillet. Add the burgers & cook with the lid closed for around 5 minutes before the bottom is browned, and the only juices apparent are no longer red. Do not put the burgers away or shift them around. Flip over and cook on medium for 3 minutes, or until cooked as needed. Take the burgers of f the flame. Let the burgers take a few minutes to rest before serving. Tip: Serve with marinara sauce on the side. Enjoy!

Nutrition:
Calories: 278
Fat: 20g
Carbs: 0.9g
Protein: 21g

46. Mexican-Style Pork Tacos

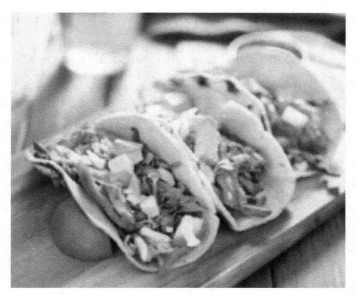

Preparation Time: 10mins
Cooking Time: 10mins
Total time: 20mins
Serves: 4

Ingredients:

- 4 tbsp of sour cream
- 6 ounces of ground pork
- 4 ounces of ground turkey
- Sea salt and ground black pepper, to taste
- 1 tbsp of lard
- 4 tbsp of tomatillo salsa roasted

- 12 lettuce leaves
- 4 tbsp of chopped cilantro

Method:
Mix black pepper, salt and pork in a bowl. Melt lard in a pan and cook meat for around 6 minutes in pan. Crumble and add tomatillo sauce. Stir and make tacos by dividing salsa mixture Between leaves of lettuce. Top with sour cream and cilantro.

Tip: Serve these wraps right away after preparing, or they will lose the tenderness. Enjoy!

Nutrition:
Calories: 330
Fat: 26. 3g
Carbs: 4.9g
Protein: 17.9g

47. Tasty Grilled Chicken Wings

Preparation Time: 2 hours and 10mins
Cooking Time: 15mins
Total time: 2 hours and 25mins
Serves: 5

Ingredients:

- Salt & black pepper as per taste
- 2 pounds of wingsJuice from one lime
- 1 handful chopped cilantro
- 2 minced garlic cloves
- 1 chopped jalapeno pepper
- 3 tbsp of coconut oil

Method:
Add all the ingredients to a bowl and toss chicken in it. Place in fridge for around 2 hours and cook each side on a preheated grill over moderate heat for around 7 minutes.
Tip: Serve with ranch dip and lime wedges on the side. Enjoy!

Nutrition:
Calories: 132
Fat: 5g
Carbs: 4g
Protein: 12g

48. Pesto Chicken

Preparation Time: 5mins
Cooking Time: 15mins
Total Time: 20mins
Serves: 1

Ingredients:

- 1/2 tsp of Black Pepper crushed
- 1 boneless Chicken Breasts
- 70 g pine nuts
- 3 tbsp of extra virgin Olive oil
- 1 cup of basil leaves loosely packed
- 2 cloves of Garlic
- 1/2 tsp of Salt
- 1/2 cup of coriander leaves loosely packed

Method:
Process all the ingredients in a blender and blitz to grind the nuts for around 30 seconds. Add one tbsp of oil and process for another 30 seconds. Marinate the chicken by putting it in a resalable bag with marinade. Place in fridge for around 1 hour and thaw before cooking. Warm a grill pan over low flame and add 1 tsp of oil. Place chicken and cook each side for around 5 minutes.
Tip: Insert the knife to check if the chicken is cooked properly. If it does not slide easily, cook for 2 more minutes. Enjoy!

Nutrition:
Calories: 300
Fat: 12g
Carbs: 7g
Protein: 10g

49. Simple and Fast Pork Chops

Preparation Time: 10mins
Cooking Time: 15mins
Total time: 25mins
Serves: 4

Ingredients:

- 1 tbsp of chopped chives
- 4 pork loin chops
- 1 tsp of Dijon mustard
- 1 tbsp of Worcestershire sauce
- 1 tsp of lemon juice
- 1 tbsp of water
- Salt & black pepper as per taste
- 1 tsp of lemon pepper
- 1 tbsp of ghee

Method:
Mix Worcestershire sauce with water, lemon juice and mustard in a bowl. Warm ghee in a pan and add pork. Add seasonings on pork and cook each side for around 6 minutes. Transfer to a plate. Simmer mustard sauce in the pan and pour over pork.
Tip: Sprinkle chives on pork and serve. Enjoy!

Nutrition:
Calories: 132

Fat: 5g
Carbs: 1g
Protein: 18g

50. Roasted Beef

Preparation Time: 10mins
Cooking Time: 8 hours
Total time: 8 hours and 10mins
Serves: 8

Ingredients:

- 1/4 tsp of dry mustard
- 5 pounds of beef roast
- Salt & black pepper as per taste
- 1/2 tsp of celery salt
- 2 tsp of chili powder
- 1 tbsp of avocado oil
- 1 tbsp of sweet paprika
- A pinch of cayenne Pepper
- 1/2 tsp of garlic powder
- 1/2 cup of beef stock
- 1 tbsp of minced garlic

Method:
Warm oil in a pan and brown each side of beef in it. Add all the ingredients except garlic and beef stock in a bowl and mix. Add roast and rub it with the mixture. Transfer to crockpot and add garlic, and stock over it. Cook for around 8 hours on low setting. Transfer to plates and serve.
Tip: Pour the juices from the crockpot over the meat before serving. Enjoy!

Nutrition:
Calories: 180
Fat: 5g
Carbs: 5g
Protein: 25g

Conclusion

For many people, a keto diet can be a healthy choice, but the ratio of fat, carbs, and protein required can vary from person to person.

If you are diabetic, discuss the diet with your doctor before beginning, as it will likely involve medication adjustments and increased blood sugar control.

On High blood pressure medication? Consult with your doctor before you continue a keto diet again.

If you are breastfeeding, don't continue a keto diet.

Be aware that restricting carbs will, among other possibilities, make you feel irritable, hungry, and tired. That, however, may be a temporary effect.

Do remember your diet should be healthy, so you get all the vitamins and minerals you need. Enough fiber is also essential.

Ketosis happens when the body starts extracting energy from stored fat rather than glucose.

Most people can safely seek out the keto diet. Nonetheless, it is best to talk to a dietitian or doctor about any significant changes to the diet. This is basically the case for those with disabilities underlying it.

A successful treatment for people with drug-resistant epilepsy could be the keto diet.

While the diet can be ideal for people of any age, children, and people over the age of 50, and infants may enjoy the greatest benefits as they can easily adhere to the diet.

Adolescents and adults, such as the modified Atkins diet or the low-glycemic index diet, can do better on a modified keto diet.

A health care provider should track closely; whoever is using a keto diet as a medication.

A doctor and dietitian are able to monitor the progress of a person, prescribe medications, and test for adverse effects.

Don't miss out!

Visit the website below and you can sign up to receive emails whenever Kimberly Thayer publishes a new book. There's no charge and no obligation.

https://books2read.com/r/B-A-NNTU-VIYAC

BOOKS 2 READ

Connecting independent readers to independent writers.

CPSIA information can be obtained
at www.ICGtesting.com
Printed in the USA
BVHW091652131022
649382BV00015B/681